Keto Meal Prep 2019:
The Complete Beginner's Guide to Save Time, Eat Healthy, and Lose Weight!

Melissa Jones

© 2019

Table of Contents

Lamb Rogan Josh

Plum Pork

Chili Orange Shrimp

Pork Stir Fry

Beef Stew

Tuna Casserole

Chicken & Mushroom Casserole

Easy Meat Loaf

Shrimp Tuscany

Easy Meatballs

Sausage & Squash Casserole

Sea Bass

Sauerkraut with Bratwurst

Roasted Chicken with Spaghetti Squash

Snacks & Vegetables

Smoked Salmon Dip

Chocolate Bacon

Guacamole

Introduction

This book should be able to help you to reach your weight loss goals! The keto diet is a great way to meet your fitness and weight loss goals, but you don't want it to consume your life. That's where meal prepping comes in handy. Meal prepping allows you to free up your schedule and still get the healthy, delicious recipes you get.

A Deeper Look at Keto

If you don't already know, this chapter will help you to get acquainted with the ketogenic diet. It causes ketones to be produced by your liver, which shifts your body's metabolism from using glucose as the primary source of fuel and instead it moves it to using fat as the main energy source. To do this, you have to restrict your intake of carbs to below a certain level, which is usually less than 100 grams a day. However, the exact amount will depend on your fitness and weight loss goals. Most people stick with less than twenty-five net carbs per day.

How It Works

Food is your body's energy source, and sadly the typical diet is a carb heavy one. That's why your body is used to using glucose as the main source of energy. The glucose is then converted to energy but also produces insulin during this process so that your body can process the glucose. Fats are then stored. With the ketogenic diet you have to deprive your body of the glucose it needs so it has no choice but to use fats instead, which allows you to enter into a state called ketosis.

Ketosis is a state that your body goes in that your liver breaks down fats instead of carbs and glucose. The ketones that are then produced are burned by the body, and you want to stay in this metabolic state. All you need to do is to follow this diet. Your calories should be 70-75% fat, 20-25% protein, and only 5-10% carbs. You may be wondering what's wrong with having more protein. To put it simply, it will affect the blood sugar and insulin in your body. When you consume protein in large quantiles, then gets converted to glucose, which will ruin your ketosis.

Ketogenic Side Effects

Most of the side effects that are related to the ketogenic diet are temporary, so you don't need to worry. These symptoms can also be called the "keto flu" because it will pass, but it isn't always pleasant. As long as you state in the state of ketosis, most if not all symptoms should be gone within a week or two.

Bad Sleep

Your body will exhibit signs when you're in the state of ketosis. You may have increased thirst, bad breath, a strong urine smell, and a loss of appetite. Your body is already in ketosis after a good night's sleep of eight hours or more because you have fasted for that long. Though, if your body isn't used to being deprived beforehand, you may start to have a restless night's sleep when you enter ketosis the first few times. Some people use vitamins supplements to help to remedy the problem due to the lowered serotonin and insulin levels. If you need a quick fix for a

restless night, you have a half a tablespoon
of fruit spread.

Digestive Issues

When you suddenly change your diet, you
may experience digestive issues including
constipation or diarrhea. The high intake of
fiber is something your body probably isn't
used to, so you may want to introduce them
slowly if the symptoms get too bad. If it
continues, then introduce fermented foods to
introduce good bacteria back into your gut to
aid in the digestive system.

Bad Breath

Bad breath may also be a sign that you just
started on your ketogenic journey. It's
completely natural, and you may notice a
fruity or metallic taste. You may even notice
a nail polish remover like odor, which is a
by-product of the acetone that's building up.
It can also be because your mouth is dryer.
It's a normal side effect, and it will pass after
your body gets used to it. If you're

socializing, then you'll want to try a non-sugar drink or piece of gum as a quick fix.

Loss of Appetite

You may lose your appetite because of your increase of fat intake. This is because you are taking in more fiber filled vegetables, fats, and nutrients that are leaving you sated. This is one of the main benefits of the ketogenic diet! A loss of appetite means that you have one less thing to worry about, so don't sweat it!

Increased Thirst

Fruit retention is natural when you're consuming carbs, but once they're flushed out by the body your water weight gets lost too. This is counterbalanced by dehydration, which is your body's way of telling you that you need to increase your water intake. Your body doesn't have water reserves when you don't have stored carbs. Drink plenty of water, and you'll be just fine.

Other Possible Side Effects

Of course, there are some other side affects you should look out for including lethargy, confusion, irritability and nausea. After about a week, you should notice these symptoms lessening or disappear altogether. Leg cramps are also common due to a loss of magnesium. Heart palpitations are also common if you allow yourself to become dehydrated due to the ketogenic diet.

The Benefits of Meal Prepping

Meal prepping is meant to make your life easier, especially when you're already using the ketogenic lifestyle to meet your health and fitness goals. In this chapter, we'll go over how meal prepping can benefit you.

It Saves Time

Meal prepping helps you to save time, so you won't be left scrambling for dinner or breakfast in the morning! Even lunch is taken care of, and sometimes left overs can even double as snacks, such as the case with pastries. When you don't have to take time every day to prep for meals, you will have more time do what you love. Your weeknights can be spent with family and friends, and you won't have to slave away in the kitchen. Once meal prepping becomes second nature, you can even schedule one day a week to dedicate to it.

It Saves Money

Meal prepping means you no longer have to buy expensive meals when you're on a crunch for time. You'd also be surprised how much you waste food because it goes bad. When you label your food and freeze it to keep leftovers you're going to use everything that you buy. This saves you more than just time but money too.

Better Portion Control

When you already have your meals made, then you have them portioned out too. This will keep you from overeating, which can help further your health and fitness goas. It can also help you to keep your drive for keto living up!

Less Unhealthy Decisions

When you have to get up to make everything you make every time you want to eat, then you're more likely to make unhealthy decisions and break your ketogenic diet. With meal prepping you can say goodbye to drive through and cheap junk food. You already have your food taken care of.

A Look at Meal Prepping & Storage

While the ketogenic diet is helpful. It can be time consuming. That's why it's important to learn how to meal prep. In this chapter, we'll go through some of the basic principles of meal prepping to help you reach your goals and free up more of your time. The goal is to have already-prepped meals in your fridge for freezer so they're easy to grab and go or simply reheat.

Keep it Simple

Make sure that you keep it easy, which means staying away from extravagant meals. Just use basic ingredients, and make sure that you store everything properly. As you get better with meal prepping, you can attempt more complicated meals.

Batch Cooking

You aren't saving time if you aren't batch cooking. The stress of cooking every single meal can be too much. Make sure that you plan ahead before you start cooking, and cook more than one meal at a time. Each recipe should serve at least four people so that you have at least four singular meals to fall back on. The more things you can cook at once, the better your meal prepping is going. Therefore, you may want to cook something that is done in the oven while cooking one that's done on top of the stove.

Storage Containers

You'll need the right containers to get started. The proper containers are essential to keeping your food as fresh as possible. You already know that you need airtight containers, but let's go over some other basics as well.

- **BPA Free:** This is a chemical found in some plastics, and it can seep into your beverages or food. BPA exposure can cause mental health issues, increase blood pressure, or even have negative effects on infants, children and even fetuses.

- **Stackable:** This is incredibly important if you're short on space. Stackable containers will help you to keep your cupboards organized. If you can stack them on top of each other in the fridge or freezer, that's a bonus too.
- **Glass Containers:** This environmentally friendly material is safe at various temperatures, allowing you to reheat your food a lot easier. Glass will cost more than plastic, but they are much more durable in the long run. Glass also won't hold the smell of your food after you've cleaned it.
- **Dishwasher Safe:** While this isn't a requirement, it can make your life a lot easier to have containers you can just throw in your dishwasher to clean.
- **Freezer Safe:** There will inevitably be times that you have to freeze the food you cook for the following week. Trying to figure out which container is and isn't freezer safe will just result in frost bitten food, so make sure that your containers are safe to throw in the freezer whenever you want.

- **Microwave Safe:** This also makes heating up your food much easier! This is another reason to go with glass if you can afford it.

A Note on Plastic Containers

If you decide to go with plastic, just make sure they're lightweight, stack easy, and are able to be frozen or microwaved. They aren't biodegradable, but they are a cheaper way to get into meal prepping. You can always upgrade your containers later. Make sure that you get BPA free plastic for your own health.

Other Storage Alternatives

There are some other containers you can use as well, including Mason Jars. Canning is a great way to store most foods, but you can use them to store salads, salad dressings, and other foods, including pudding. If you want to use Mason jars, try wide mouth jars so that it's easy to clean. Stainless steel containers are also an alternative to plastic, and they will remaining hot and cold temperatures well. Steel containers are obviously durable, but they are an expensive option. The downside of steel containers is that you cannot reheat your food in the microwave when you use these.

Always Label

It's important that you always label the food that you are putting in both your fridge and freezer. Make sure that you write down when you purchased it or the day you prepared it. This will help you to realize when food is fine to eat and when you should toss it. You become more aware of what's in your fridge so you're likely to save money and waist less too. One of the cheapest and easiest ways to label your food is a roll of freezer tape along with a permanent marker.

A Word on Thawing

If you're trying to defrost food, then place them in the fridge to thaw. However, this means you have to think in advance. You can also use cold water to thaw your food, but you have to pay more attention to it. Make sure to place your food in a leak proof bag and submerge it in cold water for thirty minutes. It should be thawed enough to reheat as desired.

Actually Reheating

Microwaving is one of the most convenient ways for you to reheat your food, and it's the quickest too. Reheat your food in one minute intervals and keep a close eye on it. Stir frequently to make sure that the temperature is even all the way through. You can also use the grill or oven to reheat your food. Although, you can also use the skillet to reheat your food over medium heat.

Two Week Meal Plan

With this two-week meal plan you'll be able to eat healthy, delicious keto friendly meals without having to cook every single day. If you have extra servings, just remember to freeze them and label them properly.

Day 1

Breakfast: Raspberry Scones

Lunch: Creamy Chicken Soup

Dinner: Keto Pot Roast

Day 2

Breakfast: Raspberry Scones

Lunch: Green Soup

Dinner: Pork Stir Fry

Day 3

Breakfast: Green Eggs

Lunch: Creamy Chicken Soup

Dinner: Lamb Rogan Josh

Day 4

Breakfast: Green Eggs

Lunch: Cobb Salad

Dinner: Keto Pot Roast

Day 5

Breakfast: Raspberry Scones

Lunch: Cobb Salad

Dinner: Sauerkraut with Bratwurst

Day 6

Breakfast: Cheddar Pancakes

Lunch: Green Soup

Dinner: Chili Orange Shrimp + Cobb Salad

Day 7

Breakfast: Chia Granola

Lunch: Cobb Salad

Dinner: Keto Pot Roast

Day 8

Breakfast: Breakfast Pudding

Lunch: Pork Burrito Bowl

Dinner: Tuna Casserole

Day 9

Breakfast: Chia Granola

Lunch: Salmon Salad

Dinner: Sauerkraut with Bratwurst

Day 10

Breakfast: Breakfast Pudding

Lunch: Pork Burrito Bowl

Dinner: Chili Orange Shrimp + Salmon Salad

Day 11

Breakfast: Cheddar Pancakes

Lunch: Salmon Salad

Dinner: Tuna Casserole

Day 12

Breakfast: Mocha Pudding

Lunch: Salmon Salad

Dinner: Tuna Casserole

Day 13

Breakfast: Raspberry Scones

Lunch: Green Soup

Dinner: Tuna Casserole

Day 14

Breakfast: Mocha Pudding

Lunch: Butternut Squash Soup

Dinner: Chicken & Mushroom Casserole

Breakfast Recipes

Raspberry Scones

Serves: 12

Time: 30 Minutes

Calories: 133

Protein: 2 Grams

Fat: 8 Grams

Net Carbs: 4 Grams

Ingredients:

- 3 Eggs, Large & Beaten   *Buy*
- ½ Cup ~~Stevia~~
- 1 ½ ~~Cups Almond Flour~~
- ~~¾ Cup Raspberries, fresh~~
- 2 Teaspoons Vanilla Extract, Pure
- 2 Teaspoons Baking Powder

Directions:

1. Start by turning your oven to 375, and then line a baking sheet with parchment paper.

BAKING sheet

2. Get out a bowl and beat your vanilla extract, stevia, eggs, baking powder and almond flour together. Fold in your raspberries, and then scoop the batter onto your pan. It should be about three tablespoons per mound, and make sure they're at least two inches apart. Bake for fifteen minutes. They should turn golden brown.

3. Transfer them to a cooling racking, allowing them to cool for ten minutes. They can be kept at room temperature for three days or in the fridge for five days or freeze for two weeks. Allow them to completely thaw before reheating.

Coconut & Cinnamon Porridge

Serves: 4

Time: 20 Minutes

Calories: 171

Protein: 2 Grams

Fat: 16 Grams

Net Carbs: 6 Grams

Ingredients:

- 2 Cups Water
- ½ Cup Coconut, Shredded & Unsweetened
- 1 Cup Heavy Cream, 36%
- 2 Tablespoons Oat Bran
- 2 Tablespoons Flaxseed Meal
- 1 Tablespoon Butter
- 1 Teaspoon Cinnamon
- 1 ½ Teaspoon Stevia
- Pinch Sea Salt

Directions:

1. Mix all ingredients together in a small pot, and put it over medium-low heat. Bring it to a slow boil, and stir well. Remove from heat.
2. Allow it to set for ten minutes so that it can thicken, and then store in mason jars. They can keep in the fridge for two days.

Coconut Flour Pancakes

Serves: 6

Time: 25 Minutes

Calories: 518

Protein: 13 Grams

Fat: 40 Grams

Net Carbs: 15 Grams

Ingredients:

- 1 Cup Butter, Melted & Unsalted
- 1 Cup Heavy Whipping Cream
- 8 Eggs, Large & Beaten
- 1 Teaspoon Vanilla Extract, Pure
- 1 Tablespoon Erythritol
- 1 Cup Coconut Flour
- 2 Teaspoons Baking Soda
- Pinch Sea Salt

Directions:

1. Get out a bowl and whisk your cream, eggs, vanilla and butter together.
2. Get out another bowl and whisk your baking soda, salt, coconut flour and erythritol together.
3. Mix your dry and wet ingredients together until it forms a smooth batter.
4. Get out a nonstick skillet and heat it over medium-high heat. Brush it down with melted butter, and then use ¼ cup portions to spoon your batter in.

cook for two minutes per side, and repeat until you fish the batch of batter.

5. You can store this in the fridge for five days or freeze for six months. Three pancakes is a serving.

Breakfast Tacos

Serves: 2

Time: 15 Minutes

Calories: 289

Protein: 7 Grams

Fat: 27 Grams

Net Carbs: 6 Grams

Ingredients:

- 4 Eggs, Large
- 2 Tortillas, Low Carb
- ½ Avocado, Sliced
- 4 Cilantro Sprigs, Fresh
- 1 Tablespoon Butter
- 2 Tablespoons Mayonnaise
- Sea Salt & Black Pepper to Taste
- Tabasco Sauce

Directions:

1. Get out a bowl and whisk your eggs before setting them aside. Get out a nonstick skillet and place it over medium heat. Swirl in your butter so that your pan is coated.
2. Add your egg in, and make sure they're spread out. Transfer to a bowl once it's cooked.
3. Warm your tortillas and then spread your mayonnaise on one side. Dive your eggs between two tortillas, and then add in your avocado and cilantro. Season with salt and pepper before rolling.
4. Add in your lime juice and wrap in foil. They can store in the freezer for one day.

Stuffed Breakfast Peppers

Serves: 4

Time: 1 Hour 5 Minutes

Calories: 459

Protein: 33 Grams

Fat: 34 Grams

Net Carbs: 6 Grams

Ingredients:

- 2 Red Bell Peppers, Halved Lengthwise & Cleaned Out
- ½ lb. Bulk Italian sausage
- 8 Eggs, Large & Beaten
- 4 Ounces Mushrooms, Sliced
- ¼ Cup Heavy Whipping Cream
- 1 Teaspoon Italian Seasoning
- Pinch Red Pepper Flakes
- ½ Cup Parmesan Cheese, Grated
- Sea Salt & Black Pepper to Taste

Directions:

1. Start by heating your oven to 4000, and then get out a rimmed baking sheet. Put your peppers on it with the cut side up, baking for five minutes. They should soften.
2. Get out a large skillet and heat up your sausage over medium-high heat, crumbling with a spoon. It should be browned after about five minutes.
3. Add in your mushrooms, cooking for five minutes. You'll need to stir occasionally.

4. Get out a bowl and whisk your cream, Italian seasoning, red pepper flakes, eggs, salt and pepper together. Fold in your mushrooms and sausage.
5. Pour this mixture into your pepper halves, sprinkling with cheese.
6. Place them in the oven cooking forty minutes.
7. Allow it to cool before storing. It'll keep in the fridge for five days or the freezer for six months.

Bacon Ricotta Muffins

Serves: 6

Time: 1 Hour 5 Minutes

Calories: 440

Protein: 27 Grams

Fat: 29 Grams

Net Carbs: 15 Grams

Ingredients:

- 2 Eggs, Large
- 1 lb. Ricotta Cheese
- 7 Ounces Bacon

- 10 Ounces Baby Spinach, Rinsed & Drained
- 2 Ounces Pine Nuts, Toasted & Chopped
- 1 Cup Parmesan Cheese, Grated Fresh
- ½ Cup Greek Yogurt, Plain
- Sea Salt & Black Pepper to Taste

Directions:

1. Start by turning your oven to 350, and then coat twelve muffin cups with cooking spray.
2. Fill a saucepan with water and bring it to a boil before and then add in your spinach. Blanch it for thirty minutes, and then drain well with a colander.
3. Dice your bacon and set that to the side, and then chop your spinach before adding it into the bowl. Add in the pine nuts, parmesan cheese, ricotta cheese, yogurt, eggs and bacon. Make sure it's evenly combined, and then divide it into your muffin cups.
4. Bake for another half hour, and then allow them to cool. They can keep in the fridge for up to three days or freeze for three weeks.

Breakfast Frittata

Serves: 5

Time: 40 Minutes

Calories: 392

Protein: 23 Grams

Fat: 31 Grams

Ingredients:

- 1 Cup Broccoli Florets, Chopped
- 8 Ounces Sausage, ground
- 1 Red Bell Pepper, Chopped
- 8 Eggs, Large & Beaten
- 2 Tablespoons Heavy Whipping Cream
- 2 Cups Spinach, Fresh
- Sea Salt & Black Pepper to Taste
- ½ Cup Cheddar Cheese, Shredded & Divided
- 3 Scallions, Sliced Thin
- Sour Cream for Garnish

Directions:

1. Start by heating your oven to 375, and then get out a large cast iron skillet. Place it over medium heat, cooking

your sausage for four to five minutes. It should brown. Remove it and then drain away all but a tablespoon of fat.

2. In the same skillet cook your spinach, bell pepper and broccoli for two to three minutes before adding your sausage back in. your spinach should wilt.

3. Get out a small bowl and whisk your cream and eggs before seasoning with salt and pepper. Pour this egg mixture over your vegetable and sausage mixture. Add in ¼ cup of your cheese, and stir until well combined.

4. Bake for twenty to twenty-five minutes.

5. Top with your remaining cheese and broil until it is melted and crisp.

6. Allow your frittata to cool before slicing it into five wedges. Place each in an airtight container. They will last in the fridge for up to five days or your freezer for three months.

Blackberry Egg Bake

Serves: 4

Time: 20 Minutes

Calories: 144

Protein: 8.5 Grams

Fat: 10 Grams

Net Carbs: 2 Grams

Ingredients:

- 1 Teaspoon Rosemary, Fresh & Chopped
- ½ Teaspoon Orange Zest
- ¼ Teaspoon Vanilla Extract, Pure
- 1 Teaspoon Ginger, Grated
- Pinch Sea Salt
- 1 Tablespoon Butter
- 3 Tablespoons Coconut Flour
- ½ Cup Blackberries
- 5 Eggs

Directions:

1. Heat your oven to 350, and then get out a blender. Blend all of your ingredients except your blackberries together, and then put each into a muffin cup.
2. Add the blackberries on top, and then bake for fifteen minutes. They will

store at room temperature for three days or in the freezer for up to a week.

Coconut Pancakes

Serves: 2

Time: 25 Minutes

Calories: 575

Protein: 19 Grams

Fat: 51 Grams

Net Carbs: 3.5 Grams

Ingredients:

- 4 Tablespoons Maple Syrup
- ¼ Cup Coconut, Shredded
- 1 Teaspoon Cinnamon
- ½ Tablespoons Erythritol
- 1 Tablespoon Almond Flour
- 2 Eggs
- 2 Ounces Cream Cheese

Directions:

1. Start by beating your eggs, and then add in your cream cheese and almond flour.

2. Now add in your remaining ingredients, and stir well.
3. Fry both sides of your pancakes, and then sprinkle with coconut on top. They will keep in the fridge for up to five days or in the freezer for two weeks.

Mocha Pudding

Serves: 4

Time: 35 Minutes

Calories: 257

Protein: 7 Grams

Fat: 20.25 Grams

Net Carbs: 2.25 Grams

Ingredients:

- 4 Tablespoons Cacao Nibs
- 2 Tablespoons Swerve
- 2 Tablespoons Vanilla Extract, Pure
- 110 Grams Chia Seeds
- 2/3 Cup Coconut Cream
- 4 Cups Water
- 4 Tablespoons Herbal Coffee

Directions:

1. Start by brewing your coffee with hot water, and then make sure the liquid is reduced by half. Strain your coffee and then add in your coconut cream, swerve and vanilla.
2. Add in your chia seeds cacao nibs, and then pour it into cubs. Allow it to set for thirty minutes before serving. It will keep in the fridge for three days.

Breakfast Pudding

Serves: 5

Time: 30 Minutes

Calories: 397

Protein: 7 Grams

Fat: 39 Grams

Net Carbs: 5 Grams

Ingredients:

- 2 Cans Coconut Milk, 13.6 Ounces Each & Unsweetened
- ¼ Cup Hemp Hearts

- ¼ Cup Coconut, Shredded & Unsweetened
- 3 Teaspoons Stevia
- 3 Tablespoons Flaxseeds
- 3 Tablespoons Chi Seeds
- Pinch Ground Cinnamon
- Pinch Sea Salt, Fine
- 2 Teaspoon Vanilla Extract, Pure
- ¼ Cup Almonds, Sliced

Directions:

1. Get out a saucepan and mix your coconut milk, hemp hearts, chia seeds, flaxseed, coconut, stevia, cinnamon and salt. Bring the mixture to a boil before reducing it to low to allow it to simmer. Whisk continuously until it begins to thicken. This should take eight to ten minutes for it to thicken properly.
2. Remove your pan from heat, and then add in your vanilla. Mix well before dividing it between five jars, and then top with almonds. Place the lids on, and then keep them in the fridge for up to six days.

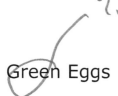

Green Eggs

Serves: 2

Time: 15 Minutes

Calories: 311

protein: 12.8 Grams

Fat: 27 Grams

Net Carbs: 4 Grams

Ingredients:

- ½ Cup Cilantro, Fresh & Chopped
- ½ Cup Parsley, Fresh & Chopped
- 1 Teaspoon Thyme Leaves
- 2 Garlic Cloves
- 2 Tablespoons Butter
- 1 Tablespoon Coconut Oil
- 4 Eggs
- ¼ Teaspoon Cayenne
- ¼ Teaspoon Cumin

Directions:

1. Start by melting your butter with coconut oil in a skillet, and then add in your garlic. Cook for a half a minute.

2. Add in your parsley, thyme, and cilantro, cooking for three more minutes.
3. Add in your eggs, and season with salt and pepper if desired. Cover, and allow it to cook for five more minutes before serving. It will last in the fridge for two days.

Breakfast Muffins

Time: 25 Minutes

Serves: 5

Calories: 364

Protein: 30 Grams

fat: 23 Grams

Net Carbs: 7 Grams

Ingredients:

- ½ Teaspoon Garlic Powder
- ½ Teaspoon Onion Powder
- 1 ½ Cups Broccoli, Chopped
- 1 Cup Ham, Cubed
- 15 Eggs, Large
- Sea Salt & Black Pepper to Taste

- ½ Cup Tomatoes, Diced
- 1 Cup Cheddar Cheese, Shredded
- 1 Teaspoon Dijon Mustard

Directions:

1. Start by heating your oven to 400, and then get out fifteen muffins cups. Silicone cups or liners can help. Spray them down with cooking spray.
2. Get out a mixing bowl and crack your eggs in. season with onion powder, garlic, salt and pepper. Whisk well, and then add in your ham, cheese, tomatoes, broccoli, and mustard. Mix well.
3. Divide your mixture into the muffin cups, making sure they're only two thirds full. Bake for fifteen minutes, and then allow them to cool. You can store them in five different containers since a serving is three muffins each. Make sure to store them in an airtight container. They'll keep in the fridge for five days, but you can also freeze them for up to three months.

Cheddar Pancakes

Serves: 4

Time: 20 Minutes

Calories: 257

Protein: 11 Grams

Fat: 24 Grams

Net Carbs; 2 Grams

Ingredients:

- 4 Egg Whites, Large
- 2 Cups Almond Meal
- 4 Tablespoons Olive Oil
- 4 Ounces Cheddar Cheese, Grated
- 1 Teaspoon Baking Powder
- 1 Tablespoon Green Onion, Fresh & Chopped

Directions:

1. Combine your cheese, green onion, garlic, almond meal and water in a bowl. Make sure it's mixed well to form your batter.
2. take your egg whites and place them in a separate bowl, mixing them with baking soda. Once it's mixed, add it

into your almond meal mixture, and beat until smooth.

3. Get out a non-stick skillet, placing it over medium-high heat, and then add in a bit of olive oil. Swirl it in your pan so that it's coasted. Ladle one eight of your batter into the skillet once it's hot, and cook for a minute per side. It should set. Continue until you use all of your remaining batter. You can keep these in the fridge for up to three days so long as they're in an airtight container.

Breakfast "Burgers"

Serves: 4

Time: 30 Minutes

calories: 504

protein: 24 Grams

fat: 41 Grams

Net Carbs: 10 Grams

Ingredients:

- 8 Portobello Mushroom Caps

- ¼ Cup Breakfast Sausage
- 4 Tablespoons Olive Oil
- 8 Ounces American Cheese

Directions:

1. Start by rinsing your mushrooms caps. You need to remove the gills and stems, and then blot them dry using paper towels before setting them to the side.
2. Get out a cast iron skillet, placing it over medium heat. Once it's hot, add in a quarter of your oil, swirling the pan until it's well coated.
3. Add in two of your mushroom caps, cooking for five minutes per side. They should be browned all over. Repeat with your remaining two.
4. Divide your breakfast sausage up into four patties, and then wipe the skillet clean, reheating it over medium heat. Add in half of your remaining olive oil, making sure your pan is coated. Cook for two to three minutes per side. It should be cooked all the way through.
5. add in your cheese on each patty, allowing it to melt.

6. Place your patties between your mushroom caps. To store these, wrap them in foil and keep them in the fridge for three days. Alternatively, you can freeze them for three weeks.

Chia Granola

Serves: 4

Time: 45 Minutes

Ingredients:

- 4 Tablespoon Flaxseed Meal
- ¼ Cup Water
- 1 Cup Macadamia Nuts
- 56 Grams Whey Protein Powder
- 4 Tablespoons Whole Chia Seeds
- 3 Tablespoons Water
- 4 Tablespoon Coconut Oil, Melted
- 4 Teaspoons Stevia
- 2 Teaspoon Cinnamon
- 1 Teaspoon Vanilla Extract, Pure
- ¼ Teaspoon Sea Salt, Fine

Directions:

1. Start by heating your oven to 350, and then get out a baking sheet. Line it

with parchment paper, and then place it to the side.

2. Get out a bowl and mix your water, chia seeds and vanilla together. Place the bowl to the side for five minutes. It should become gelatinous.

3. Place your macadamia nuts into your food processor along with your stevia, salt, cinnamon, flaxseed meal and protein powder. Pulse until it's ground up.

4. pour your chia seed mixture in next, and then add your coconut oil with a tablespoon and a half of water. Blend until it's smooth, and then set this mixture to the side. Transfer this mixture on a prepared baking sheet by the tablespoon, and then bake for fifteen minutes.

5. Remove it from the oven, and then break it up into small pieces. Spread it out before cooking for another ten minutes.

6. Pace it on a cooling rack, and then store in an airtight container for up to a week.

Lunch Recipes

Creamy Chicken Soup

Serves: 4

Time: 35 Minutes

Calories: 325

Protein: 14 Grams

Fat: 28 Grams

Net Carbs: 7 Grams

Ingredients:

- 1 Yellow Onion, Diced
- 2 Cups Chicken Broth
- 1 Cup Chicken Breasts, Cooked & Diced
- ½ Cup Water
- ½ Cup Celery, Sliced
- ¼ Cup Olive Oil
- ¼ Cup Carrot, Diced
- Sea Salt to Taste
- Herbs de Provence

Directions:

1. Get out a saucepan and place it over medium heat. Add in your oil.
2. Once your oil begins to shimmer add in your celery, carrot and onion. Cook until your onion turns translucent. Add in your nuts and chicken broth.
3. Allow it to simmer before reducing the heat. Simmer until your carrot is tender.
4. Take it off of heat and allow it to cool before blending with an immersion blender.
5. Add in ½ a cup of water and stir well. Turn the heat to medium, and stir in your chicken. Cook until reheated. This will keep in the fridge for three days or freeze for up to two weeks.

Butternut Squash Soup

Serves: 4

Time: 35 Minutes

Calories: 136

Protein: 2 Grams

Fat: 12 Grams

Net Carbs: 8 Grams

Ingredients:

- ½ lb. Butternut Squash, Cubed
- 1 Bay Leaf
- 2 Cloves Garlic, Minced
- 2 Cup Chicken Broth
- ¼ Cup Heavy Cream
- 2 ½ Tablespoons Olive Oil
- ½ Teaspoon Sea Salt

Directions:

1. Start by getting out a saucepan and heating up a half a tablespoon of olive oil over medium heat. Stir in your butternut squash and add in your garlic. Cook for five minutes, and make sure that it's lightly toasted.
2. Add in your chicken broth and remaining olive oil. Add in your bay leaf and bring your mixture to a boil. Reduce it to simmer, and simmer for twenty minutes. Your squash should be completely tender.
3. Discard your bay leaf and turn the heat off to allow it to cool. Blend using an immersion blender and pour in your cream. Blend until smooth, and reheat.

Salt before serving. It will keep in the fridge for three days or freeze for two weeks.

Green Soup

Serves: 6

Time: 35 Minutes

Calories: 392

Protein: 5 Grams

Fat: 38 Grams

Net Carbs: 7 Grams

Ingredients:

- ¼ Cup Coconut Oil
- 2 Cloves Garlic, Minced
- Sea Salt & Black Pepper to Taste
- 1 Cup Coconut Milk
- 4 Cup Vegetable Stock
- 1 Cup Watercress
- 2 Cups Spinach
- 1 Bay Leaf
- 1 Onion, Chopped
- 1 Head Cauliflower, Chopped

Directions:

1. Grease a pan with oil and cook your onion and garlic. Add in your cauliflower and bay leaf, cooking for another five minutes.
2. Add in your watercress and spinach, cooking until your spinach wilts. Add in your vegetable stock, and allow it to come to a boil. Cook for another eight minutes.
3. Add in your coconut milk, and remove it from heat. Blend until it's smooth and creamy. It will keep for five days in the fridge or it will keep in the freezer for two weeks.

Vegetable Wraps

Serves: 4

Time: 10 Minutes

Calories: 20

Protein: 0 Grams

Fat: 0 Grams

Net Carbs: 5 Grams

Ingredients:

- 1 Cucumber
- 1 Red Onion
- 1 Celery Stalk
- Dressing of Your Choice
- 2 Carrots
- 1 Head of Romaine Lettuce

Directions:

1. Slice your carrots, red onion, celery and cucumber into thin sticks, and divide between twelve lettuce leaves.
2. Drizzle with dressing and roll them up to serve. These will not freeze, but you can keep them in the fridge for up to four days.

Easy Pork Salad

Serves: 4

Time: 45 Minutes

Calories: 1050

Protein: 13 Grams

Fat: 55 Grams

Net Carbs: 5 Grams

Ingredients:

- 1 Pear, Sliced
- 2/3 Cup Blue Cheese
- 1 lb. Pork Belly, Sliced
- 4 Tablespoons White Wine Vinegar
- 4 Tablespoon Olive Oil
- 1 Teaspoon Mustard
- 2 Teaspoons Water
- 2 Tablespoons Stevia
- 2/3 Cup Walnuts, Chopped
- 4 Teaspoons Sea salt, Fine
- 4 Cups Salad Leaves

Directions:

1. Take half of your oil and cover your pork. Cook at 350 for a half hour.
2. Warm up a pan and add in your water and stevia. Stir until your stevia dissolves, and then add in your walnuts. Cook for five minutes. Allow your nuts to cool, and then chop your pear and cheese into bite size pieces.
3. Make the dressing by adding in your remaining oil, mustard and vinegar together.

4. Take your pork out of the oven, and cut into bite size pieces. Toss all ingredients together rand drizzle with your dressing before serving. It can last in the fridge for three days.

Pork Chili

Serves: 8

Time: 4 Hours 15 Minutes

Calories: 466

Protein: 31 Grams

Fat: 36 Grams

Net Carbs: 4 Grams

Ingredients:

- 2 lb. Pork Shoulder, Boneless & Cubed
- 1 Onion, Chopped
- 3 Tablespoons Chili Powder
- 1 Teaspoon Garlic Powder
- 1 Teaspoon Ground Cumin
- 1 Teaspoon Coriander
- 1 Teaspoon Sea Salt, Fine
- 1 Cup Sour Cream
- 1 Cup Cheddar Cheese, Shredded

Directions:

1. Get out a slow cooker and combine the onion, pork shoulder chili powder, garlic powder, cumin and salt. Mix well, and allow it to cook on high for four hours.
2. Allow it to cool and then ladle a cup and a half of the chili into eight storage containers. Garnish with cheese and sour cream only before serving. It will store for six months in your freezer or five days in your fridge.

Pork Burrito Bowls

Serves: 4

Time: 4 Hours 35 Minutes

Calories: 528

Protein: 41 Grams

Fat: 35 Grams

Net Carbs: 12 Grams

Ingredients:

- ½ Avocado Oil, Divided

- 1 Bunch Cilantro, Fresh & Chopped
- 3 Limes, Juiced
- 1 Jalapeno Pepper, Minced
- 6 Cloves Garlic, Minced
- 6 Scallions, Minced Fine
- ½ Teaspoon Sea Salt, Fine
- 1 lb. Pork Belly
- 1 Onion, Sliced
- 2 Cups Cauliflower Rice, Cooked
- 1 Green Bell Pepper, Sliced Thin
- 1 Cup Cheddar Cheese, Shredded
- ½ Cup Sour Cream
- 1 Avocado, Halved, Pitted & Chopped

Directions:

1. Get out a medium bowl and whisk your lime juice, jalapeno, salt, garlic, cilantro and ¼ cup of your oil together. Add in your scallions but keep two tablespoons of the mixture set aside.
2. Add your remaining mixture into a zipper top bag and then add in your pork belly. Coat until it's marinated, and then seal your bag. Refrigerate for four hours but no more than eight hours.

3. Get out a skillet, placing it over medium-high heat and adding in your remaining oil.
4. Once your oil shimmers, wipe off any excess marinate from your meat, and cook in the hot oil for about five minutes per side. Set it aside.
5. Add your onion and bell pepper to the same skillet, and cook for five minutes. Your vegetables should be soft.
6. Slice your meat thin, and then return it to the pan. Add in your reserved marinade, and cook while stirring for two minutes.
7. Divide your vegetable and meat mixture with your cauliflower rice between four containers. It'll keep for five days in the fridge.

Salmon Salad

Serves: 4

Time: 10 Minutes

Calories: 446

Protein: 34 Grams

Fat: 31 Grams

Net Carbs: 9 Grams

Ingredients:

- 3 Scallions, Chopped Fine
- 3 Dill Pickles, Chopped Fine
- 8 Ounces Flaked Salmon, Fresh or Canned
- ½ Cup Mayonnaise
- 1 Teaspoon Dijon Mustard
- 3 Tablespoons Olive Oil
- 1 Lemon, Juiced & Zested
- 1 Teaspoon Dill
- Black Pepper to Taste

Directions:

1. Get out a large bowl and combine your pickles, salmon and scallions. Get out another bowl and whisk together your zest, juice, dill, pepper, mustard, mayonnaise and oil.
2. Mix both mixtures together, and divide between storage containers. It will keep in the fridge for up to five days.

Balsamic Salmon Salad

Serves: 4

Time: 35 Minutes

Calories: 456

Protein: 36 Grams

Fat: 34 Grams

Net Carbs: 7 Grams

Ingredients:

- 4 Salmon Fillets, 4-6 Ounces Each
- 2 Tablespoons Olive Oil
- Sea Salt & Black Pepper to Taste
- 1 Tablespoon Coconut Oil
- ½ Cup Whole Pecans
- 1 Tablespoon Erythritol
- ¼ Cup Raspberries, Fresh
- 4 Cups Salad Greens, Mixed
- ¼ Cup Feta Cheese, Crumbled

Directions:

1. Get out a baking sheet and line it with foil. Preheat your broiler to high. Rub each fillet down with olive oil before seasoning with salt and pepper.

2. Place it in the oven, cooking for eight to twelve minutes. The salmon should flake with a fork. Set it to the side.
3. Get out a skillet and place it over medium heat, adding in your coconut oil, erythritol and pecans. Stir constantly while cooking for three to five minutes before removing from heat. Your erythritol should be dissolved.
4. Get out a large bowl and mix together your feta, greens and berries.
5. Divide evenly between storage containers. It'll keep in the fridge for up to four days.

Easy Chili

Serves: 5

Time: 6 Hours 25 Minutes

Calories: 629

Protein: 46 Grams

Fat: 37 Grams

Net Carbs: 15 Grams

Ingredients:

- 8 Ounces Ground Beef, Cooked & Drained
- 8 Ounces Bacon, Uncured, Diced, Cooked & Drained
- 1 Cup Beef Broth
- 8 Ounces Ground Sausage, Cooked & Drained
- 1 Cup Celery, Chopped
- 15 Ounces Canned Diced Tomatoes, In Juice
- 6 Ounces Tomato Paste, Canned
- 4 Ounces Green Chilies, Canned & Diced
- 1 Tablespoon Worcestershire Sauce
- 1 Tablespoon Chili Powder
- 1 Tablespoon Ground Cumin
- 1 Teaspoon Garlic Salt
- 1 Teaspoon Ground Black Pepper
- Shredded Cheese to Garnish
- Sour Cream for Garnish

Directions:

1. Get out a slow cooker and add in all of your ingredients. Stir until well combined, and then cook on high for four to six hours.

2. Allow it to cool beef dividing it up, topping with shredded cheese and sour cream to serve. It's best to top with sour cream after you reheat it. It will keep in the fridge for five days or in the freezer for three months.

Caesar Salad

Serves: 4

Time: 10 Minutes

Calories: 586

Protein: 33 Grams

Fat: 50 Grams

Net Carbs: 6 Grams

Ingredients:

- ¾ Cup Caesar Dressing
- 1 Cup Grape Tomatoes
- 4 Eggs, Hard Boiled & Sliced
- ½ Cup Red Onion, Sliced Thin
- 2 Cups Baked Chicken Thighs, Cooked & Boneless
- ½ Cup Parmesan Cheese, Grated
- 1 Romaine Lettuce Head, Chopped

Directions:

1. Get out four Mason Jars, and then place three tablespoons of your dressing at the bottom. This is so that your salad doesn't get soggy.
2. Layer with the remaining ingredients, and shake before serving. They will last in the fridge for up to four days.

Cobb Salad

Serves: 4

Time: 20 Minutes

Calories: 545

Protein: 33 Grams

Fat: 38 Grams

Net Carbs: 10 Grams

Ingredients:

- 2 Romaine Lettuce Heads, Chopped
- 2 Cups Chicken Thighs, Baked, Boneless & Chopped
- 1 Cup Grape Tomatoes
- 2 Cucumbers, Diced

- ½ Cup Red Onion, Chopped
- 4 Slices Bacon, Cooked & Chopped
- ½ Cup Ranch Dressing, Dairy Free
- 4 Hard Boiled Eggs, Sliced
- ½ Cup Blue Cheese, Crumbled

Directions:

1. Divide your lettuce leaves between four storage containers, and then distribute the rest of your ingredients except for your dressing into each one.
2. Divide your dressing by two tablespoons and then store it on the side. If you store it together, your salad will get soggy.
3. Make sure that your containers are air tight, and they'll keep in the fridge for up to five days.

Beef & Cabbage Stir Fry

Serves: 4

Time: 35 Minutes

Calories: 550

Protein: 49 Grams

Fat: 33 Grams

Net Carbs: 8 Grams

Ingredients:

- 1 Tablespoon Coconut Oil
- 1 ½ lbs. Ground Beef
- 2 Cloves Garlic, Minced
- 1 Green Cabbage Head, cored & Chopped
- 2 Tablespoons Apple Cider Vinegar
- 2 Tablespoons Coconut Aminos
- Sea Salt & Black Pepper to Taste
- 4 Scallions, Fresh & Chopped
- Toasted Sesame Oil Seeds to Garnish
- Sriracha to Garnish
- Sesame Seeds to Garnish

Directions:

1. Start by heating your olive oil using medium heat in a large skillet. Cook your garlic and beef until your beef is browned, which should take five to seven minutes.
2. Add in your cabbage, cooking for eight to ten minutes. It should be slightly wilted.
3. Next add in your vinegar, coconut amnions, salt and pepper.

4. Divide between four containers. Top with srirarcha, toasted sesame oil, scallions and sesame seeds just before serving.
5. When storing your meal, it'll last up to five days in the fridge.

Dinner Recipes

Easy Pork Chops

Serves: 4

Time: 30 Minutes

Calories: 481

Protein: 15 Grams

Fat: 32 Grams

Net Carbs: 4 Grams

Ingredients:

- 1 Teaspoon Garlic, Crushed
- 1 Onion, Chopped
- 4 Pork Chops
- 1 Tablespoon Paprika
- ½ Cup Heavy Cream
- 1 Tablespoon Butter
- 1 Tablespoon Parsley, Chopped
- 1 Cup Mushrooms, Sliced
- 2 Tablespoons Coconut Oil
- ¼ Teaspoon Cayenne Pepper
- Sea Salt & Black Pepper to Taste

Directions:

1. Start by mixing all of your seasoning together with a third of your onion, and rub it into both sides of your pork chop.
2. Heat up some coconut oil, browning your pork chops on both sides before placing them to the side.
3. Add in your mushrooms and remaining onion, cooking for four minutes.
4. Whisk your butter and cream in the pan, and add your pork chops in. cook for five more minutes. They will last in the fridge for three days or in the freezer for two weeks.

Keto Pot Roast

Serves: 6

Time: 4 Hours 30 Minutes

Calories: 521

Protein: 69 Grams

Fat: 25 Grams

Net Carbs: 6 Grams

Ingredients:

- 2 ½ lbs. Rump Roast
- 1 Onion, Small
- 1 Clove Garlic, Large
- 1 Thyme Sprig, Fresh
- 1 Turnip, chopped
- 1 ½ Cups Beef Stock
- 1 Cup Radishes, Halved
- 2 Tablespoons Heavy Cream
- 1 ½ Tablespoons Olive Oil
- Sea Salt & Black Pepper

Directions:

1. Start by setting your oven to 475, and then season your pork using salt and pepper.
2. Get out a Dutch oven and place it over high heat, adding in your olive oil. Make sure it's coasted, and then brown your roast on all sides.
3. Set your roast to the side, and sauté your onion until browned, and then add it to your roast.
4. Add in your garlic, thyme and beef stock. Return your roast and onion mixture back in and then add in your radishes and turnips. Place it

uncovered in the oven at 400, and cook for four to five hours.

5. Allow it to cool before placing your vegetables in a bowl.

6. Get out a saucepan, placing it over medium heat and add some liquid from your Dutch Oven. Stir in your heavy cream, and allow it to come to a boil. Reduce the heat to a simmer, and then slice your pot roast thin.

7. Divide between containers, and serve with vegetables and sauce. It will keep in the fridge for up to three days.

Lamb Rogan Josh

Serves: 6

Time: 4 Hours 10 Minutes

Calories: 450

Protein: 38 Grams

Fat: 28 Grams

Net Carbs: 4 Grams

Ingredients:

- 1 ½ Kg Lamb, Diced

- 1 Cup Greek Yogurt, Plain
- 2 Tablespoons Ghee
- Rogan Josh Curry Paste
- 2 Red Onions, Sliced
- Sea Salt & Black Pepper to Taste

Directions:

1. Start by mixing all ingredients together, and add in some water. Simmer for four hours. It will keep in the fridge for three days or in the freezer for two weeks.

Plum Pork

Serves: 8

Time: 4 Hours 10 Minutes

Calories: 316

Protein: 24 Grams

Fat: 20 Grams

Net Carbs: 10 Grams

Ingredients:

- 1 Tablespoon Allspice
- 1 Tablespoon Cinnamon

- 1 Cup Bouillon
- 2-3 lbs. Pork Belly
- 4 Plums, Chopped

Directions:

1. Slice into the skin on your pork so that the flavor soaks through. Rub your pork down with cinnamon and allspice.
2. Mix all of your remaining ingredients into a sauce, and then put the pork back in the pot. stew for four hours.
3. This will keep in the fridge for five days or can last in your freezer for three weeks.

Chili Orange Shrimp

Serves: 4

Time: 15 Minutes

Calories: 186

Protein: 28 Grams

Fat: 6 Grams

Net Carbs: 3 Grams

Ingredients:

- Pinch Cinnamon
- 1 Chipotle Chili
- 1 Teaspoon Orange Zest
- 1/8 Teaspoon 5 Spice
- Sea Salt & Black Pepper to Taste
- 2/3 Cup Cream
- 2.5 lbs. Shrimp, Peeled & Deveined

Directions:

1. Start by blending your cream, chili, orange and salt and pepper together.
2. Add it into the frying pan with your shrimp, and season with the remaining ingredients.
3. Sauté for five minutes before serving. It will keep in the fridge for three days or your freezer for one week.

Pork Stir Fry

Serves: 6

Time: 25 Minutes

Calories: 698

Protein: 54 Grams

Fat: 50 Grams

Net Carbs: 4 Grams

Ingredients:

- 3 Tablespoons Coconut Oil
- 1 lb. Ground Pork
- 6 Scallions, Sliced
- 2 Cups Green Cabbage, shredded
- 1 Tablespoon Ginger, Fresh, Peeled & Grated
- 3 Garlic Cloves, Minced
- 2 Lime, Juice
- 1 Tablespoon Soy Sauce
- ½ Teaspoon Chili Oil
- ½ Teaspoon Sesame Oil

Directions:

1. Get out a skillet and heat up your coconut oil over medium-high heat. Once your oil shimmers, add in your pork and cook for five minutes. It should start to brown.
2. Add in your scallions, ginger and cabbage. Cook while stirring often for three minutes. Add in your garlic, and cook for half a minute.
3. Add in your soy sauce, sesame oil, chili oil and lime juice. Cook for one to two more minutes.

4. Divide between six containers. It will last either in your freezer for six months or your fridge for three days.

Beef Stew

Serves: 8

Time: 4 Hours 15 Minutes

Calories: 933

Protein: 69 Grams

Fat: 66 Grams

Net Carbs: 6 Grams

Ingredients:

- 1 ½ lb. Chuck Roast, Cubed
- 2 Red Onions, Chopped Roughly
- 1 lb. Button Mushrooms, Halved or Quartered
- 8 Ounces Pearl Onions, Frozen
- 1 Cup Red Wine, Dry
- 4 Celery Stalks, Chopped Roughly
- 2 Teaspoon Garlic Powder
- 1 Teaspoon Thyme
- 1 Teaspoon Rosemary
- 1 Teaspoon Sea Salt, Fine

- ¼ Teaspoon Black Pepper
- 1 Tablespoon Dijon Mustard

Directions:

1. Get out your slow cooker and combine your mushrooms, red onions, beef, pearl onions, celery, wine, garlic powder, thyme, rosemary, mustard, salt and pepper. Stir well, and then cook on high for four hours.
2. Allow it to cool before placing it in eight containers. It will keep for five days in the fridge or six months in your freezer.

Tuna Casserole

Serves: 9

Time: 1 Hour 30 Minutes

Calories: 761

Protein: 53 Grams

Fat: 59 Grams

Net Carbs: 9 Grams

Ingredients:

- ¼ Cup Avocado Oil
- 1 Onion, Chopped
- 2 Zucchinis, Sliced
- 3 Cloves Garlic, Minced
- 1 lb. Tuna, Oil Packed & Drained
- 1 Cup Cheddar Cheese, Shredded
- 1 Tablespoon Dijon Mustard
- 1 Teaspoon Dill
- 1 Lemon, Zested
- 1 Can Cream of Mushroom Soup

Directions:

1. Start by heating your oven to 350, and then get out a nonstick skillet. Add in your oil, placing it over medium-high heat. Once your oil begins to shimmer, add in your onion and zucchini. Cook while occasionally stirring for five minutes. Your vegetables should soften.
2. Add in your garlic, and stir constantly for a half a minute. Remove it from heat, allowing it to cool.
3. Get out a bowl and combine your lemon zest, dill, mustard, and soup together. Whisk until smooth before adding in your tuna, cheese and

vegetables. Make sure it's well combined.
4. Get out a nine by thirteen-inch baking dish, and bake for an hour. It should bubble.
5. It will store in the fridge for three days or keep in the freezer for six months.

Chicken & Mushroom Casserole

Serves: 8

Time: 1 Hour 15 Minutes

Calories: 609

Protein: 25 Grams

Fat: 56 Grams

Net Carbs: 9 Grams

Ingredients:

- 8 Chicken Thighs, Bone In
- 1 lb. Button Mushrooms, Halved
- 1 Cup Cheddar Cheese, Shredded
- 1 Cup Cream of Mushroom Soup, Cooled
- 8 Ounces Pear Onions, Frozen

Directions:

1. Start by heating your oven to 350, and then get out a nine by thirteen-inch baking dish.
2. Mix your onions, mushrooms and chicken thighs in the bottom of your pan, and then get out a bowl.
3. In your bowl mix your soup and cheese together before pouring it into the pan as well.
4. Bake and cover with foil for an hour and fifteen minutes. The chicken should be cooked all the way through. Allow it to cool before storing in the fridge for three days or the freezer for up to six months.

Easy Meat Loaf

Serves: 4

Time: 45 Minutes

Calories: 481

Protein: 49 Grams

Fat: 27 Grams

Net Carbs: 10 Grams

Ingredients:

- 8 Ounces Ground Pork
- 8 Ounces Ground Beef
- 1 Egg, Large
- ¼ Cup Parmesan Cheese, Grated
- ½ Cup Pork Rinds, Crushed
- ¼ Cup Heavy Whipping Cream
- 1 Teaspoons Yellow Mustard
- Sea Salt & Black Pepper to Taste
- 3 Cups Green Beans, Blanched
- 1 Tablespoon Erythritol
- 1 Tablespoon Apple Cider Vinegar
- ¼ Cup Tomato Paste

Directions:

1. Start by heating your oven to 400 before lining a baking sheet with foil.
2. Get out a bowl and combine your pork rinds, pork, beef, egg, cream, mustard and parmesan. Season with salt and pepper, and then form into a loaf shape. Place this onto your baking sheet.
3. In a bowl mix your vinegar, ketchup and erythritol. Brush on top of your meatloaf.

4. Cook for thirty-five to forty minutes. Allow it to cool before slicing into four pieces. It can store in the fridge for up to five days or last in the freezer for three months.

Shrimp Tuscany

Serves: 4

Time: 15 Minutes

Calories: 298

Protein: 23 Grams

Fat: 18 Grams

Net Carbs: 6.5 Grams

Ingredients:

- ¼ Cup Baby Kale
- 5 Tomatoes, Sun Dried
- ½ Cup Milk, Whole
- 1 Teaspoon Basil
- 1 Teaspoon Sea Salt, Fine
- ½ Cup Parmesan
- 2 Cloves Garlic, Crushed
- 1 Cup Cream Cheese
- 1 Teaspoon Butter

- 1 lb. Shrimp, Raw

Directions:

1. Start by melting your butter in a pan and then add in your shrimp. Cook for about a half a minute or until they turn pink.
2. Add in your milk and cream cheese and increase the heat. Stir and cook until the cheese melts completely.
3. Add in your salt, garlic, and basil. Bring it to a simmer, and cook until your sauce thickens.
4. Serve with kale and tomatoes, and allow to cool completely. It will store in the freezer for one week or the fridge for three days.

Easy Meatballs

Serves: 4

Time: 1 Hour 5 Minutes

Calories: 380

Protein: 25 Grams

Fat: 23 Grams

Net Carbs: 8 Grams

Ingredients:

- 1 Teaspoon Thyme
- 1 Teaspoon Oregano
- ½ Cup Mozzarella, Sliced
- 1 Can Tomatoes, Peeled
- 1 lb. Beef, Minced
- 1 Handful Basil, Fresh
- 1 Tablespoon Tomato Paste
- 2 Cloves Garlic, Crushed
- ½ Cup Red Onion, Diced

Directions;

1. Heat your oven to 350, and then get out a bowl. Mix your beef and herbs together before forming sixteen meatballs.
2. Fry them in a skillet over medium-high heat for five minutes to brown them, and set some of the cooking juices to the side.
3. Add in your onion, tomatoes, tomato paste and garlic. Allow them to simmer for ten more minutes. Put your meatballs in a dish, and break up your cheese before spreading it over the sauce.

4. Cook in the dish while covered with foil for twenty minutes.
5. Take the foil off and bake for five more minutes. They will store in the fridge for five days or your freezer for two weeks.

Sausage & Squash Casserole

Serves: 10

Time: 1 Hour

Calories: 402

Protein: 31 Grams

Fat: 24 Grams

Net Carbs: 15 Grams

Ingredients:

- 1 Spaghetti Squash, Large
- 1 Onion, Minced
- ½ lb. Turkey Sausage
- ½ lb. Italian Sausage
- ½ lb. Ground Beef, Lean
- ½ lb. Mushrooms, Sliced
- 18 Ounces Tomatoes, Diced
- 8 Ounces Parmesan Cheese, Grated

- 4 Ounces Mozzarella Cheese
- 6 Ounces Tomato Paste
- ½ Cup Butter
- ½ Cup Red Wine
- 4 Ounces Ricotta Cheese
- Sea Salt & Black Pepper to Taste

Directions:

1. Start by setting your oven to 350, and then pierce your spaghetti squash with a sharp knife, and then microwave on high for twenty minutes. Set it to the side to cool.
2. Get out a skillet, placing it over medium-high heat to melt your butter. Sauté your ground beef and sausages until they're browned, crumbled and cooked all the way through. Add in your red wine, and allow it to simmer until your liquid reduces. Stir in your garlic and onion, sautéing until tender. Add in your mushrooms, and sauté until tender.
3. Add in your diced tomatoes and remaining seasonings. sauté for three to four more minutes.
4. Halve your squash and scrape out the flesh before setting it to the side.

5. Spread half of your spaghettis squash into a baking dish and then add two ounces of mozzarella and two ounces of ricotta. Top it off with four ounces of parmesan, and then spoon tomato sauce over it before adding the remaining squash. Add remaining cheeses, and bake covered for twenty minutes.
6. Uncover and bake for an additional twenty minutes.
7. Set your oven to a broil for three minutes.
8. Allow it to cool for fifteen minutes before slicing. It will keep in the fridge for five days, and it will keep in the freezer for two weeks.

Sea Bass

Serves: 4

Time: 25 Minutes

Calories: 380

Protein: 27 Grams

Fat: 26 Grams

Net Carbs: 3.4 Grams

Ingredients:

- 4 Lemons, Divided
- 2/3 Cup Green Olives
- 2 Cups Cauliflower, Grated
- 2 Seabass
- 2/3 Cup Parsley, Fresh & Chopped
- 2/3 Cup Mint, Fresh & Chopped
- Sea Salt & Black Pepper to Taste

Directions:

1. heat your oven to 400, and then get out a baking pan. Line it with parchment paper, and then put your fish on top.
2. Rub your fish down with olive oil and slice your lemons. Stuff into the bass along with your herbs and bake for fifteen minutes.
3. In the meantime, chop up your olives and juice your other lemons. Take the bowl and mix together all remaining ingredients.
4. Serve your fish topped with your remaining ingredients. This will keep in the fridge for three days or the freezer for one week.

Sauerkraut with Bratwurst

Serves: 4

Time: 50 Minutes

Calories: 525

Protein: 24 Grams

Fat: 42 Grams

Net Carbs: 8 Grams

Ingredients:

- 2 Tablespoons Avocado Oil
- 1 Yellow Onion, Sliced Thin
- 1 lb. Bratwurst
- 16 Ounce Jar of Sauerkraut, Drained
- 1 Teaspoon Garlic Powder
- 1 ½ Cups Chicken Broth
- Sea Salt & Black Pepper to Taste

Directions:

1. Start by getting out a large cast iron skillet before adding in your oil, placing it over medium heat. Add in your bratwurst and onion, cooking for six to eight minutes.

2. Add in your broth, garlic powder, salt, pepper and sauerkraut. Simmer for thirty to forty minutes. Your sausage should be cooked all the way through.
3. Split into four portions in different airtight containers. It will last in the fridge for up to five days, and it will last in the freezer for three months.

Roasted Chicken with Spaghetti Squash

Serves: 4

Time: 45 Minutes

Calories: 361

Protein: 18 Grams

Fat: 30 Grams

Net Carbs: 6 Grams

Ingredients:

- 1 Teaspoon Garlic Powder
- 1 Teaspoon Onion Powder
- 1 Prepared Spaghetti Squash
- ¼ Cup Pesto Sauce
- Sea Salt & Black Pepper to Taste

- ¼ Cup Olive Oil
- 3 Chicken Thighs, 3-4 Ounces Each, Bone In

Directions:

1. Start by heating your oven to 375, and then get out a shallow dish. Pat your chicken thighs dry using paper towels before placing them in the dish.
2. Add in your garlic, onion, oil, salt and pepper. Make sure that your chicken is coated evenly.
3. Put your chicken on a baking sheet, and bake for thirty to forty minutes. Your chicken should be cooked all the way through.
4. Get out a medium bowl and toss your spaghetti squash with pesto sauce, seasoning with salt and pepper. Make sure it's well coated.
5. Divide your squash noodles and chicken between four containers. In the fridge it will keep for up to six days. In the freezer it will keep for three months.

Snacks & Vegetables

Smoked Salmon Dip

Serves: 8

Time: 15 Minutes

Calories: 70

Protein: 5 Grams

Fat: 5 Grams

Net Carbs: 2 Grams

Ingredients:

- 4 Ounces Smoked Salmon
- 4 Ounces Cream Cheese, Full Fat
- 2 ½ Tablespoons Mayonnaise
- 2 Tablespoons Dill, Fresh & Chopped
- Sea Salt & Black Pepper to Taste

Directions:

1. Mix all ingredients together in a food processor, pulsing until well combined. Season with salt and pepper.

2. It will keep in the fridge for up to three days, and you can serve it with cucumber sticks, celery or carrots.

Chocolate Bacon

Serves: 6

Time: 20 Minutes

Calories: 258

Protein: 7 Grams

Fat: 26 Grams

Net Carbs: 0.5 Grams

Ingredients:

- 12 Bacon Slices
- 4 ½ Tablespoons Dark Chocolate, Unsweetened
- 1 ½ Teaspoons Liquid Stevia
- 2 ¼ Tablespoons Coconut Oil

Directions:

1. Start by heating the oven to 425, and then skewer your bacon using iron skewers. Spread it out, and then bake for fifteen minutes. It should become

crispy. Allow your bacon to cool completely.
2. Get out a saucepan and melt your coconut oil over low heat, and stir in your chocolate until it's melted.
3. Add in your liquid stevia, and make sure it's well combined.
4. Put your bacon on parchment paper, and coat in chocolate on both sides. Allow it to dry before storing in an airtight container. It will keep for five days in the fridge.

Guacamole

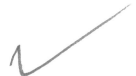

Serves: 6

Time: 15 Minutes

Calories: 172

Protein: 2 Grams

Fat: 15 Grams

Net Carbs: 11 Grams

Ingredients:

- 3 Avocados, Large
- 1 Red Onion, Diced

- 4 Tablespoons Lime Juice
- ½ Teaspoon Cayenne Pepper
- Sea Salt & Black Pepper to Taste

Directions:

1. Halve your avocados, discarding the stone before scooping the flesh out into a large bowl. Mash well, and then add in your remaining ingredients.
2. Store in the fridge for three days and serve with celery, carrot or cucumber sticks.

Parmesan & Walnut Bites

Serves: 10

Time: 50 Minutes

Calories: 80

Protein: 7 Grams

Fat: 3 Grams

Net Carbs: 7 Grams

Ingredients:

- 6 Ounces Parmesan Cheese, Grated
- 2 Tablespoons Walnuts, Chopped

- 1 Tablespoon Butter, Unsalted
- ½ Tablespoons Thyme, Fresh & Chopped

Directions:

1. Start by heating your oven to 350, and then get out two rimmed baking sheets. Line with parchment paper before placing your baking sheets to the side.
2. Get out a food processor and combine your butter and parmesan.
3. Pour in your walnuts, continuing to pulse until they're crushed and combined.
4. Scoop the mixture onto your baking sheets by the tablespoon and top with thyme.
5. Bake for eight minutes. They should be golden brown.
6. Allow them to cool for a half hour before storing in an airtight container. They should last in your fridge for five days.

Eggplant Spread

Serves: 8

Time: 15 Minutes

Calories: 54

Protein: 2 Grams

Fat: 4 Grams

Net Carbs: 4 Grams

Ingredients:

- 1 lb. Eggplant
- 2 ½ Tablespoons Roasted Red Peppers, Chopped
- 2 Tablespoons Pine Nuts
- 2 Tablespoons Olive Oil
- ½ Tablespoon Feta Cheese, Crumbled
- 1 Tablespoon Lemon Juice, Fresh
- Garlic Powder to Taste
- Sea Salt & Black Pepper to Taste

Directions:

1. Heat your oven to 400, and then slight your eggplant lengthwise, arranging it on a baking sheet with baking paper.
2. Roast your eggplant for an hour. It should become tender. Allow it to cool

before scraping the eggplant from the skin, adding it to your food processor. Add in your remaining ingredients, and except for your feta cheese, and pulse until smooth.

3. Sprinkle with feta cheese, and fold it into the mixture. It will keep in the fridge for up to five days. It's best served with celery, cucumber sticks or carrots.

Collard Greens

Serves: 5

Time: 6 Hours 10 Minutes

Calories: 82

Protein: 5 Grams

Fat: 2 Grams

Net Carbs: 2 Grams

Ingredients:

- 1 – 1 ½ lbs. Collard Greens, Chopped
- 1 Bay Leaf
- 1 Onion, Chopped
- 3 Tablespoons Balsamic Vinegar

- 1 Tablespoon Olive Oil
- 1 Tablespoon Garlic, Minced
- 2 Cups Vegetable Stock

Directions:

1. Throw your onions into your slow cooker, cooking on high for five minutes.
2. Add in your remaining ingredients, and cook on low for six hours. It will store in the fridge for five days, or you can freeze it for two weeks.

Stuffed Portobello Mushrooms

Serves: 6

Time: 1 Hour

Calories: 239

Protein: 16 Grams

Fat: 17 Grams

Net Carbs: 12 Grams

Ingredients:

- 6 Portobello Mushrooms Caps, Large
- 2 Eggs, Small

- 3 Garlic Cloves, Minced
- 1 ¼ Cup Ricotta Cheese, Full Fat
- ¾ Cup Spinach, Steamed
- ¾ Cup Parmesan Cheese, Grated
- ½ Cup Olive Oil
- Sea Salt & Black Pepper to Taste

Directions:

1. Start by heating your oven to 425, and then get out a baking sheet. Line your baking sheet with foil.
2. Start by rinsing your mushroom caps until all the dirt is gone. Discard your stems and gills, and blot them dry using paper towels.
3. Season with salt and pepper, and then place them on a baking sheet. Bake for fifteen minutes.
4. While your mushroom caps are baking, combine your remaining ingredients well in a bowl before setting it to the side.
5. Take your mushroom caps out of the oven and fill them with your mixture. Bake for an additional twenty-five minutes. They should be tender and heated all the way through. Allow them to cool before storing. They will keep in

the fridge for three days. It is not recommended that you freeze them because it can lose texture.

Ham & Green Bean Salad

Serves: 6

Time: 30 Minutes

Calories: 102

Protein: 4 Grams

Fat: 8 Grams

Net Carbs: 5 Grams

Ingredients:

- 1 lb. Green Beans, Trimmed
- 2 White Onions, Minced
- 2 Roasted Red Bell Peppers, Diced
- 2 Ounces Spanish Ham, Chopped
- 2 Hardboiled Eggs, Chopped
- 5 Tablespoons Flat Leaf Parsley, Fresh
- 4 Tablespoons Olive Oil
- 3 Tablespoons Red Wine Vinegar
- Sea Salt & Black Pepper to Taste

Directions:

1. Rinse your green beans and drai before steaming them. Blot them with a paper towel before putting ...em to the side.
2. Get out a bowl and combine your vinegar, olive oil, salt and pepper. Make sure it's mixed well.
3. Mix your green beans with ha, peppers, onion, egg and parsley. Divide between serving bowls and add in your dressing.
4. Cover and keep in the fridge for two days.

Spicy Coleslaw

Serves: 4

Time: 5 Minutes

Calories: 103

Protein: 2 Grams

Fat: 7 Grams

Net Carbs: 11 Grams

Ingredients:

- 4 Cups Green Cabbage, Shredded

- 6 Scallions, Chopped Fine
- 1 Bunch Cilantro, Fresh & Chopped
- ¼ Cup Apple Cider Vinegar
- 1 Lime, Juiced
- ½ Cup Avocado Oil
- ½ Teaspoon Sriracha
- ½ Teaspoon Chinese Hot Mustard
- 1 Clove Garlic, Minced
- 1 Tablespoon Sesame Seeds
- 1 Teaspoon Ginger, Fresh, Peeled & Grated
- ½ Teaspoon Sea Salt, Fine

Directions:

1. Get out a bowl and combine your cilantro, scallions and cabbage. Mix well, and then get out a bowl.
2. Whisk your oil, vinegar, sriracha, lime juice, sesame seeds, mustard, garlic, salt and ginger together.
3. Get out four containers, and place a cup into each. Add in three tablespoons of your dressing, and toss well. It will keep for five days in the fridge, but you can't freeze it.

Caprese Salad

Serves: 4

Time: 10 Minutes

Calories: 373

Protein: 25 Grams

Fat: 28 Grams

Net Carbs: 6 Grams

Ingredients:

- 12 Ounces Mozzarella Cheese, Fresh & Chopped
- ¼ Cup Olive Oil
- ½ Teaspoon Sea Salt, Fine
- 1/8 Teaspoon Ground Black Pepper
- 1 Bunch Basil Leaves, Fresh & Chopped
- 3 Tomatoes, Large & Chopped

Directions:

1. Get out a bowl and combine everything together. Make sure it's mixed well, and then keep it in the fridge for up to three days. This cannot be frozen.

Cauliflower Mash

Serves: 4

Time: 30 Minutes

Calories: 143

Protein: 3 Grams

Fat: 14 Grams

Net Carbs: 3 Grams

Ingredients:

- 1 Cauliflower Head
- ¼ Cup Butter, Unsalted & Melted
- 1/8 Teaspoon Ground Black Pepper
- ½ Teaspoon Sea Salt, Fine
- ¼ Cup Heavy Whipping Cream

Directions:

1. Break your cauliflower into florets and then place them in a pot, covering them with water. Bring it to a boil over medium-high heat, and cook for ten minutes.
2. Drain, and then mash them. Stir in your remaining ingredients.

3. Divide between four storage containers and store in the fridge for five days or freeze for six months.

Healthy Jalapeno Poppers

Serves: 8

Time: 35 Minutes

Calories: 240

Protein: 12 Grams

Fat: 20 Grams

Net Carbs: 3 Grams

Ingredients:

- 6 Ounces Cream Cheese, Room Temperature
- ½ Cup Pepper Jack Cheese, Shredded + Some Reserved for Garnish
- 16 Jalapeno Peppers, Halved & Deseeded
- 8 Slices Bacon, Cooked & Crumbled

Directions:

1. Start by heating your oven to 350, and then get out a bowl. Mix your cream cheese and pepper jack cheese together, spooning this mixture into your jalapenos.

2. Put them with the cheese side up on a rimmed baking sheet before topping with bacon and your reserved cheese.

3. Bake for twenty-five minutes, and then place them into eight containers. It will last for five days in the fridge.

Green Bean Casserole with Cheese

Serves: 4

Time: 25 Minutes

Calories: 366

Protein: 15 Grams

Fat: 31 Grams

Net Carbs: 12 Grams

Ingredients:

- 3 Cups Green Beans, Cooked
- 2 Cups Cream of Mushroom Soup
- ½ Cup Cheddar Cheese, Shredded
- ½ Cup Caramelized Onions

Directions:

1. Start by heating the oven to 350, and then get out a bowl. Mix your beans, soup, onion and cheese together.
2. Get out a nine by thirteen-inch baking dish, and spread your mixture in it. Bake while uncovered for fifteen minutes.
3. Store for up to five days in the fridge.

Caramelized Onions

Yields: 2 Cups

Time: 30 Minutes

Calories: 63

Protein: 1 Gram

Fat: 2 Grams

Net Carbs: 8 Grams

Ingredients:

- ¼ Cup Avocado Oil
- 4 Onions, Sliced Thin
- 1 Teaspoon Sea Salt, Fine

Directions:

1. Start by getting a skillet over and heat your oil over medium-high heat.
2. Once it shimmers add in your salt and onion. Stir and cook for twenty to thirty minutes.
3. Split between four containers, and then keep them in the freezer for six months or the fridge for five days.

Caramelized Onion Dip

Serves: 6

Time: 30 Minutes

Calories: 211

Protein: 4 Grams

Fat: 18 Grams

Net Carbs: 8 Grams

Ingredients:

- ¼ Cup Avocado Oil
- 2 Onions, Sliced Thin
- ½ Teaspoon Sea Salt, Fine
- 1 Teaspoon Thyme
- 8 Ounces Cream Cheese, Room Temperature

- 1 Teaspoon Dijon Mustard
- 2 Red Bell Peppers, Sliced
- ¼ Cup Mayonnaise

Directions:

1. Get out a nonstick skillet and heat up your oil over medium-high heat. It should shimmer.
2. Reduce the heat to medium-low before adding in your salt, thyme and onions.
3. Cook while stirring for twenty to thirty minutes. Allow it to cool before coming with your mayonnaise, mustard, cream cheese and onions together. Mix well, and it will keep in the fridge for up to three days.

Spinach Stuffed Mushrooms

Serves: 8

Time: 35 Minutes

Calories: 162

Protein: 9 Grams

Fat: 13 Grams

Net Carbs: 4 Grams

Ingredients:

- 8 Ounces Cream Cheese, Room Temperature
- 4 Ounces Spinach, Frozen & Thawed, Wrung Out & Chopped
- 1 Teaspoon Dijon Mustard
- 1 Teaspoon Garlic Powder
- 2 Dashes Tabasco Sauce
- 1 Tablespoon Shallot, Minced
- ½ Cup Parmesan Cheese, Grated
- 1 lb. Button Mushrooms, Stemmed

Directions:

1. Start by heating your oven to 425, and then get out a bowl. Mix your spinach, mustard, cream cheese, garlic powder, shallot, parmesan and Tabasco.
2. Put your mushrooms on a baking sheet, and make sure the cap side is down. Spoon your mixture into each cap, and bake for twenty-five minutes.
3. It will keep in the fridge for up to five days.

Spicy Deviled Eggs

Serves: 12

Time: 10 Minutes

Calories: 72

Protein: 3 Grams

Fat: 6 Grams

Net Carbs: 3 Grams

Ingredients:

- 6 Hard Boiled Eggs, Peeled & Halved Lengthwise
- ½ Cup Mayonnaise
- 1 Dill Pickle, Minced
- 1 Teaspoon Dijon Mustard
- 2 Scallions, Minced
- 1 Clove Garlic, Minced
- 1/8 Teaspoon Cayenne Pepper
- ½ Teaspoon Sea Salt, Fine

Directions:

1. Scoop your yolks out and place them in a bowl. Put the whites on a platter with the cut side up.
2. Mix your yolks with the remaining ingredients, and mix until mashed and well combined.
3. Pipe into your egg halves, and then store in the fridge for up to five days.

Brussel Sprouts & Bacon

Serves: 4

Time: 30 Minutes

Calories: 347

Protein: 16 Grams

Fat: 26 Grams

Net Carbs: 10 Grams

Ingredients:

- ¼ Cup Avocado Oil
- ½ Teaspoon Sea Salt, Fine
- 1/8 Teaspoon Ground Black Pepper
- 4 Ounces Bacon, Chopped
- 1 ½ lbs. Brussel Sprouts, Halved Lengthwise
- 4 Ounces Bacon, Chopped

Directions:

1. Start by heating your oven to 400, and then get out a bowl. Toss your sprouts, bacon, salt, pepper and oil together.
2. Get out a rimmed baking sheet, placing your sprouts on them. Cook for

twenty minutes, but turn them halfway through.
3. Divide between four containers, and they will keep in the fridge for up to five days. Freezing them can cause a texture issues.

Conclusion

The ketogenic diet doesn't' have to be hard, and with meal prepping it won't be. All you need is to pick a few recipes to get started, or follow the meal plan provided to get started! You don't have to cook every day, and most people can choose to just cook all of their meals once or twice a week, giving you more free time to enjoy your life while sticking to your health goals. A healthy lifestyle should become second nature, and ketogenic meal prepping is the first step towards that.

More in <u>The Melissa Jones Collection</u>, found at Amazon.com!

So.   Noel.
          app-

6/25/19-
BENZONATATE 100 my caps
(Generic for Tessalon Perless
1 Caps 3 times a day as needed for
                                cough
                         742- 2700
2 3 4/08/0/3/3   04553995

very eathy throat
      &
cough - continued

Flour - white -
Flour - wheat
oil - " soda /
Baking powder - ½ tsp
sooji - ½ cup -
oil - 2 tblsp
buttermilk -

oil for frying

Let it covered
& let it
for 1 Hour
cover - damp
cloth

/

PART - white flour - 1 part
        wheat " - 3 " (2.3 cup
Baking powder
curd (over night →) leam
salt - 1 teasp
oil, ghee or Butt -
⅓ / ½ cup H_2O
oil for frying.

¾ cup dahi, ½ tablesp sugar
½ teasp Baken powder
¾ cup all purpose
¼ " H_2O (optional)

Made in the USA
San Bernardino, CA
28 February 2019